FITNESS

Nutrition, Exercises, and Body Building

Johnny Fitness

TABLE OF CONTENTS

Johnny Fitness

Introduction

Trying to embrace a healthy diet in order to lose weight is hard enough even if you were not exercising. You have to count calories, watch what you eat and do lots of other lifestyle transformations in order to live the life of the new you who wants to lose weight and keep the weight off. Well, much as this is important, it doesn't have to be as difficult as many people seem to put it. You don't need to engage in strenuous physical activity that you hate, eat veggies all the time and make other sacrifices that you are never ready to make.

With the right exercise, you can actually lose weight, keep it off and live a healthy, disease free life. You won't need to worry about not eating your favorite foods even if it is once in a while. When you look forward to a fat burning exercise, you can indulge in that cake and be sure to burn it in your next session – or better still, pay it forward and get in the exercise first, then you can feel all virtuous as you tuck in.

This book will provide you with several workout exercises that you can try out today as well as workout tips to know where you may have been going wrong with your workouts in the past. It will also help you to make your workouts effective so that you can start losing weight and looking and feeling healthier.

Chapter 1

Work Out Exercise and Tips to Lose Weight

Walking/Running

One of the easiest ways to burn calories and lose weight is walking or running, depending on where you are as far as your weight is concerned. If you are slightly heavier, you should stick to walking, as it has been proved that the risk of injuries to the knees or causing other stress-induced injuries to your body are less, so it is safer that way. Additionally, walking/running improves your mental wellbeing. Furthermore, walking at a speed of four miles per hour will burn between 5 and 8 calories every minute, or between 225 and 360 calories for a 45-minute walk. This is to say that if you walked at this pace for 45 minutes a day, you will be able to lose up to a pound a week in weight, which is the healthy way to do it.

The convenience that walking/running has to offer is immeasurable. The fact that there is no equipment that is required and that you do not need a gym membership for you to be successful at it, makes it the perfect exercise. However, what happens when you are not in a position to do your workout outside for whatever reason; bad weather, safety reasons and so on? The treadmill could be your best friend.

The Treadmill

Although it is true that nothing beats working out outside with the fresh air, the inspiring scenery, and the company of other people among other reasons that make working out outside seem so delightful, the truth of the matter is that it at times proves impossible for you to work out from outside for various reasons. So, when your options are limited, the good old treadmill takes over.

Weight loss and the treadmill go hand in hand. The reason behind the working of treadmills is they simulate real-life movement, to be specific running and walking depending on which stage of activity you are at. These simulations are a great way to burn calories and thus lose weight. Treadmills are therefore a very good way to lose weight if it so happens that you do not have a safe space to run or walk outside.

In order to enjoy the maximum benefits of a treadmill, here are some important tips to bear in mind.

Tips For Working Out On The Treadmill To Lose Weight

Make sure you do not hold the sidebars

When you are on the treadmill, you should bear the entire weight of your own body; therefore you should ensure that you do not hold onto the handles of your treadmill as you walk or run. When you carry your own weight as you walk, you burn more calories as opposed to leaning on the treadmill where some of the strain that should be carried by your feet is taken up by the bars of the treadmill. The proper way in which you carry your weight is seen in the figure below.

Keep up with the treadmill speed

Keep pace with the speed of the treadmill so that you do not rest or 'take it easy'. This will give you a better workout and also avoid accidental falls.

Use the incline feature of the treadmill

Ensure that you are making use of the calorie-zapping incline feature that allows you to pick up intensity in your workout without necessarily breaking into a run. When walking on an inclined treadmill, walk normally as you would up a hill outdoors. In addition, the way you place your feet on the treadmill also matters and you should let your feet come down underneath your center of gravity as opposed to them being far out in the front.

The figure below shows the inclined/slanted feature on the treadmill where you set it so that you are able to pick up intensity just as you would when running up a hill.

Choose appropriate exercise shoes

When choosing exercise shoes, you should always keep in mind that wearing the wrong kind of shoes on a treadmill could be fatal. This is not just scaremongering. Slipping and falling on the treadmill does not only lead to broken bones, it could and has led to deaths. Make sure that you buy shoes with extra padding on the soles. This offers protection to your heels and foot bones from the high impact of your mass as you take a stride or rather a step.

Place your foot on the treadmill properly

When you land your foot flat on the treadmill while exercising on it, chances are that you will end up with muscle strain. This is because you end up leaning backward when the treadmill belt moves forward, which in turn strains the muscles due to the force that is generated throughout your hips and back. Losing your balance is also not out of the question if you are not careful how you place your foot on the treadmill belt. Always ensure you are perfectly vertical so that you can run as you would normally do on real ground. Landing on your mid-foot or the part known as the ball of your foot (not your heel) ensures you are exercising safely. See photo below.

Use the right posture on the treadmill

Leaning on the treadmill in any direction leads your body to naturally work hard to maintain balance. This is a strain no one needs while exercising. Hunching forward while walking on the treadmill could make you suffer a back tilt or cause you to lose your balance and may contribute to lower back pain. Keeping a solid upright posture that involves your core muscles is advisable to avoid unnecessary pain. Whenever you are unable to maintain an upright posture, make sure you slow down your speed on the treadmill.

Place your arms appropriately

Swinging your arms round while working out, or winging them out to the sides or even crisscrossing as you walk is not efficient. What happens is that you end up burning up a lot of energy with your arms, and you end up not being able to work out as long as you should. Keeping your arms by your sides until you get to higher speeds really helps you get the best results from working out on the treadmill. Once you have reached the jog stage, ensure that you keep your arms bent parallel to each other and at 90-degrees, but loose. This will help with the rotation of your torso. Check the image below.

Do not make extra long strides

You might assume that when you take long strides, you are covering more ground as opposed to someone taking shorter strides. The truth of the matter is that long strides end up sacrificing form and efficiency. The only thing that you will end up doing is that you will burn up a lot of extra energy so that you cannot workout as long as you really should. Long strides also increase the risk of injuries in that you could easily hit the front of the treadmill frame, which would inevitably lead to a fall. The standard way to run on a treadmill is normally three steps per second, making sure that you barely lift your foot off the ground.

Avoid the urge to look at your feet or lose concentration

As unlikely as it might seem, you should be aware that looking at your feet while walking on the treadmill is very risky. In the first place, it could make you lose your balance and fall, causing injuries. It has also been shown to strain the neck and lead to misalignment of the rest of the body, resulting in your hips poking out behind you. This stresses the hips, spine and the knees. Whenever you are on the treadmill, always ensure that you gaze straight ahead and keep your shoulders level and chest open. This automatically will make your hips, knees, and low back align to follow, making a relatively straight line from your head to your feet. This is the correct way to ensure that you do not suffer strain or injuries.

Inverted V Pipe Exercise

This exercise is amazing as it works on your core, arms and lower back.

-Lie down on the floor as you face downwards. Raise your body by pushing using your hands and feet until you form an inverted V.

-Once you achieve the inverted V position, pose for a few seconds then return to the starting point.

Bent Leg Rotating Exercise

This workout works your abs and inner thigh.

-Stand straight and put your hands at the back of your head. This is usually to give you more strength and to bring concentration to your legs.

-Lift your bent right leg to your waist. While you leg is still bent, rotate it in circular movements.

-Rotate it several times like for about 15 seconds to the front and 15 seconds to the back.

-Once you are done with the right leg, move to the left leg and do the same.

Bridge Exercise

This is a very effective exercise that works your hamstrings, your abdominal region, your glutes as well as your lower back.

-Start by laying on your back then have your arms by your side.

-Bend your knees and raise your hips while ensuring that your back is straight. Let the hips be in a straight line with your knees and shoulders.

-Hold for about 30 seconds then lower your hips back to the initial position gently then repeat this for a few more minutes.

Workout Tips To Lose Weight

Sticking to one particular routine of exercise over a long time

One thing you should always be aware of is that the more you do a particular routine on the treadmill, the easier your body adapts to this same kind of exercise and your muscles becomes more efficient. You should ensure that every four weeks, you change at least one aspect of your work out. You should try the elliptical or the stair climber, or better still, take your exercising outside. Routine changes also help you prevent muscle and joint strains from repetitive stress of pulling and pushing muscles at the same angles over and over again.

Over exercising

You probably wouldn't think that there is any such thing as over-exercising, especially now when you want to lose weight desperately. Well, there is such a thing as overdoing it as far as exercise goes. Your body can only take so much activity without being given time to recuperate. Whenever you realize that you are suffering from excessive muscle soreness, elevated heart rates even when at rest, and little aches and pains that keep getting worse with each workout, these are signs that you are probably over training. For general fitness, you should ensure that you perform moderate workouts between three to five times per week. Keep in mind that high intensity workouts should be done between two to three times in a week.

Johnny Fitness

Chapter 2

Workout Exercises for Building Muscles

We all know how hard it is to actually find a workout routine to build muscle that works. Here are some tips to help you to gain those muscles. The truth is that for muscle gaining exercises, all you have to do is to stick to the basics. Here are a few ideas on how to do workout exercises that will actually build muscle.

Rest-Pause Sets

As far as muscle building goes, training volume is crucial. For your muscle to grow, putting enough stimuli is very important. Rest-pause works by basically having you perform a few repetitive racking of the weight you are lifting for about fifteen seconds and then un-racking it and continuing to work. When this is done for several sets, you will notice that you start to feel your muscles being strained. The reason why this kind of exercise works so well for muscle gain is that it allows you to get to fatigue quickly while ensuring that you also get more of the reps that 'matter'.

Always start by picking a strong exercise, preferably a heavy hitter such as back squats, bench press and so on. After you make sure that your body has been thoroughly warmed up, load the bar with weights that equates to somewhere between 3 and 5 reps, and get under the bar and perform one repetition. Take a 15 – 30 seconds rest and then do another repetition. For it to be as effective as it should be, ensure that you do up to 10 sets. Once you achieve all 10, it is advisable to increase the weight for your next session. As you are going to find out for yourself, rest-pause training is very taxing, and for this reason, it would be better to start with only one or two exercises a week and progress upwards.

The image above shows how you are supposed to exercise with a heavy hitter and perform back squats like in the second image.

The below image shows you how to perform bench press with a considerable amount of weights to get better results as far as muscle building goes.

Drop sets- Mechanical Advantage

You should be aware that your muscle system works as a series of 'levers' and 'pulleys' that move your joints during an exercise. For this reason, certain positions while exercising will definitely give your muscles an advantage to be properly exercised. For example, wide grip pull-ups are more difficult to execute than when you perform close-grip pull-ups. This is because of the position you have placed your limbs and consequently the muscles involved. How you maximize on this concept is by ensuring that you begin at your weakest position and move towards your stronger positions. As you become fatigued, you realize that your exhaustion is on a completely new level.

The wide grip pull-ups that are shown on the above are difficult to execute as opposed to the close grip-ups. Always start with a wide grip and perform as many of these as possible until you cannot do any more of them. As soon as you are done, immediately shift to a parallel grip with your palms facing each other and continue. After these are done, shift to a chin up position where you are able to grip (underhand) and crank out a few more. You should be able to do at least two to three more reps with each grip change. This is the same type of workout that you could apply to bench press and back squats.

For better results, start with one set at the end of your workout and progressively add up to three sets over the course of a few weeks.

The figure below elaborates how you start with a wide grip as you perform as many of these as possible.

Complexes

This routine helps in increasing your training density and fatigue to a particular group of muscle. Supersets are used to ensure you gain maximum advantage of this exercise. When you work three to four exercises in a row, you find that you compound a certain group of muscles to fatigue, which leads these muscles to gain an intense stimulus for them to grow.

For you to be able to incorporate complexes into your routine, what you are supposed to do is that you should select a group of muscles and then choose up to 3 for intermediate, or 4 for advanced exercises. For elaborations, the diagram below shows how you could exercise your upper body muscles through strain.

Power Exercise

Do about 3-5 repetitions of push ups, where after each push up, you clap to slow down the rate at which you execute one push up before you get into the next one. This sets the pace for your muscles to be stretched.

Strength Exercise

Doing about 6-8 repetitions of dumbbell Bench presses as shown in the figure below

Isolation Exercise

8-12 repetitions of cable chest- fly. The figure below helps you see exactly what happens.

Front Squat

Squats are among the most inclusive and basic exercises that you can do for your lower body. The front squat is an amazing muscle growth booster.

-Grasp the barbell from floor or rack with overhand open grip that is slightly wider than shoulder width. Position the barbell chest high with your back arched. Place the bar in front of your shoulders with the elbows put forward as high as you can go with fingers under bar on each side.

-With your helps slightly wider than shoulder width, position your feet outward at around 45°.

-Go down slowly until your knees are fully bent and the thighs are almost parallel to the floor. As you go down, ensure that the knees travel outward in the direction of the toes. Return and repeat the process.

Back squat

-Start from the rack with the barbell at upper chest height. Ensure the bar is high on back of shoulders then grasp the barbell to the sides.

-Remove the bar from rack and stand at shoulder width distance.

-Descend until your thighs are straight and the knees pout to the same direction as your feet. Extend your knees and hips until your legs are straight then repeat the process.

Tips for Gaining Muscle

Unlike exercising to lose weight, exercising to gain muscle is very different. Given you have been exercising for what is probably a very long time to lose weight, you might feel a bit put off upon hearing that for you to gain muscle, you have to increase your food intake. The fact that we have always heard that for you to lose weight you have to reduce the amount of food we take may have made it a taboo for you to admit that you actually want to gain weight. Well, it is also right to say that even in muscle building, we are supposed to watch the kind of food we eat. Excess carbohydrates are never good whatsoever for your body, muscle building or otherwise. So what exactly are you supposed to be doing for you to be able to gain muscle? Here is what to do.

Eat more

You must be very confused after reading this subtitle, especially since you have reduced your food portions in an attempt to lose weight. Well, what I mean by eating more here does not refer to eating excess food that has no value to your body. There is a formula you should apply for you to be able to tell if you are eating the required amount of food for your body to be able to build the muscle you are after.

Work out your biggest muscles

When you work out your body intensely especially for a beginner, your protein synthesis is bound to increase. If you have been lifting weights for a while, muscle building will be quickest if your focus is on the large group of muscles in your body such as in your legs, back and chest. This means that you need to start embracing squats, dead lifts, pull-ups, bent-over rows, bench presses, and military press-ups that help you exercise a large group of muscles.

Eat proteins

Muscle gain is all about protein intake. It does not matter how hard you exercise; if you are not taking in the proper portion of proteins, you are not going to gain the muscle that you are desperately looking for. The truth is that most lean men who do not gain muscle do not fail to gain muscle due to their wrong exercising routines, but rather it is because they are simply eating the wrong kind of food. You are supposed to eat at least a gram of protein per pound of your body weight. This amount of protein is roughly the maximum amount of protein your body can use in a day. For instance, a 160-pound man should take about 160g of proteins a day, which is the amount of protein he could possibly get from an 8-ounce chicken breast, or a roast beef sandwich, or a cup of cottage cheese, or two eggs, or a glass of milk, or two ounces of peanuts. The rest of your calories should be split between carbohydrates and fats.

Have a drink before workouts

Research has proved taking a shake containing amino acids and carbohydrates right before exercising greatly enhances protein synthesis compared to if you were to take the shake after doing the exercise. The shake should contain at least 6 grams of amino acids-the building blocks of proteins, which are responsible for muscle growth and 35g of carb. When you are working out, blood flow to your working tissues increases and the carbohydrate-protein mixture in your body encourages a greater uptake of amino acids into your muscles. The reason I would advice you to consider taking a drink instead of a solid source of these proteins and carbohydrates is because of the simple fact that liquid meals are usually absorbed faster into the body. Therefore, ensure you take a shake high in protein and carbohydrate around an hour before your workout in order to enjoy the greatest benefits after the workout.

Chapter 3

Workout Exercises and Tips to Tone Your Body

After all the weight is gone and the muscle has been built, the icing of your cake is getting your body toned in the right places for you to confidently show off that body you have worked so hard for. The following routines are going to help you with that toning process.

Squat/Chair pose

This kind of exercise targets to tone your glutes, quads, and your hamstrings.

-Start by standing with your feet apart (shoulder –width). Hold light dumbbells to your sides.

-Assume a squat position, pushing your butt behind you; keeping your body weight over your heels.

-Then push up through your heels to a standing position squeezing your glutes. Do up to 20-25 repetitions.

-After you are through with your last rep, drop the weights and bring your feet together. Resume the squat position, keeping your knees behind your toes and extend your arms in front to your chest level-hold for about 30 minutes.

You could challenge yourself as you go along with heavier dumbbells.

Chest Fly

Just as the name suggests, this exercise tones your chest and shoulders (the upper body).

-Start by laying on the ground, or a bench with your knees bent.

-Hold considerably heavy dumbbells with your arms extended and your palms facing each other. Keep your elbows slightly bent as you slowly open your arms out to the sides.

-Stop when the weights are an inch above you then push the weights to the starting position. Do 15 reps. Take the lighter sets of dumbbells and repeat this process; 10 more reps should be fine.

Plank combo/Push-Up

This is the perfect workout routine to tone your upper body (Chest and shoulders) as well as your triceps and abs.

-You can make this exercise easier by modifying your push up position. Place your palms on the ground slightly wider than your shoulders and your knees.

-Keep a straight line from the top of your head through your legs. Ensure you hold your abs in a tight position then bend your elbows 90 degrees and push back to start. Do 20 to 25 reps.

-After you are done, lift your knees off the ground so that you are in a full push up position with your legs extended. Keep your abs tight with your back straight, and then hold for thirty seconds.

Doing full push-ups and holding for about 60 seconds will lead to faster toning.

Biceps Curl

This exercise routine targets your biceps. Doing biceps curls consistently for at least a month will lead to toned upper arms.

-Start the exercise by standing with your knees slightly bent and your feet close together. Hold a heavy dumbbell in each of your hands; your palms should face up.

-Slowly curl the weights towards your shoulders in contrast to your biceps. Lower the weights slowly to your starting position and repeat the process up to 15 reps.

-Immediately, pick up lighter weights and repeat up to 10 more steps.

Plie squat

This exercise tones your inner thighs, quads and your glutes.

-Start the exercise by standing with your feet slightly wider than your shoulder-width distance and with your toes turned out. Hold lighter dumbbells vertically in front of your thighs. Keep your abs tight and your torso tall.

-Bend your knees 90 degrees, and have them aligned between second and third toes and place your weight in your heels.

-Press back the start position as you press your glutes. 15 reps should work for this routine.

Inner /Outer leg lift

This exercise tones your outer thighs, the inner thigh and your glutes.

-Stand with your feet hip-width apart.

-Extend your arms at shoulder height and have your palms down.

-Lift your left leg to the side, squeezing your outer thigh and glutes. Do up to 15 repetitions of this.

-For better results, continue by making sure that you do not touch the floor, and bring your left leg in front of your body. Rotate your inner thigh to face forward. Do up to 15 repetitions of this.

-Switch your legs and start from the beginning.

Roll up

This exercise routine tones your deep transverse and gives you what is commonly known as a six pack.

-Start by laying face up with your knees bent then extend your arms next to your ears ensuring to let your palms face up.

-Extend your arms straight in front of you while contracting your abs. Lift your head, neck and shoulders off the ground.

-Ensure that your spine is rounded, moving as smoothly as possible.

-After you are all the way up, tighten your abs and rollback down. Do up to 8 repetitions.

The side reach

This routine aims at toning your abdominals and obliques.

-Lie on the ground on your right side.

-Have your legs stacked one on top of the other.

-Your right arm should be on the ground and your left arm should be on top of your left leg.

-Pull your abs in as you move your left hand down as if you want to touch your ankle.

-Move slightly off the ground as you feel the contraction along your side.

-Move your back slowly as you make use of your obliques and abs to provide the required resistance. Do up to 8 repetitions and switch up the sides and repeat the whole process.

Boat Pose

This workout routine also tones your abs into what we call a 'six pack' as well as your deep (transverse).

-Sit on the ground with your knees bent then place your feet in a hip-width distance apart.

-Place your hands under your thighs and inhale deeply.

-Exhale as you lift your feet off the ground. You should keep your knees bent and pull your abs in tightly.

-Lean back slightly and balance on your glutes then open your arms wide out to your sides. Hold this for up to 8 breaths, return to start and repeat the entire process.

Do up to 3 repetitions of this.

Opposite arm and leg Lift

This exercise tones your lower body, upper body, triceps, biceps and glutes

-Get down on all fours with your knees under your hips and hands under your shoulders.

-Reach your right arm forward as your stretch the left leg backwards. Hold for around five seconds then release and repeat using your right leg and left arm. This is just one rep. do 10-15 reps.

Kneeling Glute toner

This exercise tones your glutes, inner and outer thighs.

-Kneel with your knees hip-width apart then hold the back of a chair; tuck pelvis and tighten abs.

-Slide your left foot back then lift knee and toes off the floor then press back straight with foot and do 20 reps.

-As your knee is still behind your hip and the pelvis tucked, turn you leg out slightly, lift toes 20 repetitions.

-Rotate your thigh out, and press your back 29 reps.

-Finally, lift the leg diagonally to the side 20 reps. Repeat the same with the other leg.

Twisting Knee Plank

This is an amazing exercise to tone your butt, lower and upper body as well as your arms.

-Get into the up part of push-up then twist the lower body to left then to right and then return to the center.

-Bring the left knee forward in order to touch your left elbow. Hold this position for a second then return to the center and do the same on the right side. This is one rep. Do 20 repetitions.

Johnny Fitness

Chapter 4

Exercising in Water

Some people have problems exercising with weights, or even exercising on land. That may be because of a number of reasons. If you are overweight, or have joint problems, it could be difficult for you to exercise effectively for as long as you need to in order to build muscle and/ or lose weight. It's not just about swimming, either, although that is an excellent all round exercise that people of all ages, weights and fitness levels can do. These are the best ways to exercise in water if you're looking to build muscle or lose weight.

Swimming

Swimming is one of the best all round exercises there is. It builds muscle, burns fat and helps you to lose weight. And you don't need any special equipment, other than a swimsuit. The big plus with swimming is that people of all ages and fitness levels can swim, because you can start slowly, and build up as you get used to it. Because the water supports your weight and your joints, even heavily overweight people or people suffering from arthritis can swim, whereas they may well be unable to cope with other forms of exercise. Any exercise is better than none at all, so even if you can only manage a few lengths of the pool at first, it's a good start towards a fitter, healthier you.

Swimmers tend to be slimmer and have more defined muscle groups than non-swimmers, and it's easy to see why this should be. A fairly gentle swim can burn around 500 calories an hour, while a more strenuous bout of water workout can dispose of 700 calories in the same time frame. You need to get rid of 3,500 calories to lose one pound of fat, so if you only have a gentle swim twice a week, that would be 52,000 calories expended in a year – or almost 15 lbs, without doing anything else at all to lose weight. A 15 lb weight loss would solve many people's weight problems, and encourage others to keep going, so swimming can be very motivational, and it's also enjoyable.

Another bonus with swimming is that, unlike many other exercises, you don't necessarily need to take rest days to protect against injuries. That's because the water cushions your body and your joints, so if you enjoy swimming and want to swim every day or most days, there's absolutely no reason why you shouldn't. You can swim for the rest of your life, and you will reap the anti-aging benefits of swimming as well as the fitness and weight loss bonuses, because swimmers tend to have lower blood pressure and blood cholesterol levels, and improved cardiovascular and brain health compared to non-swimmers.

Swimming is a complete body workout – no other form of exercise can make that claim, and it's also enjoyable. And you can swim all year round without discomfort. If you like to go running or cycling, in the hot summer months you may need to scale back a little, but with swimming, you can keep the work rate going all year round. There are so many advantages to swimming for weight loss, muscle building and fat burning that it's difficult to comprehend why everybody doesn't do it on a regular basis. And that's not the end of the story. If you can't swim, or if you want to vary your water workout, there are other ways to exercise in water.

Aqua aerobics

Aqua or water aerobics are, simply put, aerobic exercises in water. You don't need to be able to swim to take part, so if you can't swim but want all the benefits of exercising in water, maybe aqua aerobics is the answer. The main advantage of water aerobics over hitting the gym or regular, land-based exercise is that the resistance of the water means you can exercise for longer without getting weary or running the risk of injury through over exercising. That's particularly beneficial if you are overweight, unfit, or physically disabled due to arthritis or joint pain.

Muscle function and range of movement is significantly increased by exercising in water, so your workout will be much more effective than working out on land, and it's 75% less stressful on the joints, according to expert opinion. Another big plus with water exercise is that, as with swimming, you won't build up such a sweat that it makes exercising uncomfortable. That means it's easier for people with cardiovascular problems, as well as allowing for longer exercise periods during the warmer months.

In water, your body feel around 90% lighter than it actually is, so you can run and jump with ease, even if you are overweight, unfit, or have joint problems which make traditional land-based exercise difficult or even impossible. You can expect to burn between 400 and 500 calories in an hour-long session of aqua aerobics, which is excellent news if you want to lose weight.

Another consideration is the resistance in water is 12 times that of exercising on dry land. That means greatly improved muscle tone and strength, and a higher metabolism, which also helps with weight loss. It's all good news for fans of water exercise.

Water running

Just plain old running through water as opposed to running on land has many benefits. For a start, there isn't the stress on the joints. Pounding the pavements can send a shock wave equivalent to five times your weight through your body, and the buoyancy of the water can counteract that. Also, because your legs and your body have to work against the resistance of the water, you will burn double the calories if you run in water – 11 per minute, as opposed to 6 per minute running on dry land. Even walking through water burns twice the calories as walking on dry land. And you will get these benefits even if you run on the spot, standing waist-deep in water in the pool. It's not a good idea to try this in the sea though – could be dangerous if you get a freak wave.

If you want to take water running to the next level, you can try deep water running (DWR). Originally developed to help injured runners rehabilitate themselves, many athletes now use it as an integral part of their training. Deep-water running means running in water deep enough that your feet don't touch the bottom. Only your head, neck and shoulders should remain above water. Some DWR practitioners use a flotation vest, but it's not compulsory. The big advantage is that the depth of water reduces total body strain by as much as 90%, yet you still get the same cardiovascular workout you receive in regular running. And the extra viscosity of water as opposed to air actually increases the intensity of the workout.

For DWR to be really effective, you need to remember a few important factors. Keep your body as upright as possible, lift your knees higher than you would when jogging, and point your toes slightly. If you can get your knees up to your hip, that's really good going, but it may take a while to get to that stage, so don't force it. As you jog, swing your arms loosely from the shoulders, with the elbows bent and the palms of your hands clenched into a relaxed fist or turned inwards. You're aiming to move them efficiently through the water in a clean, crisp slice, not scoop it up.

Water running isn't for everyone – you may not feel confident, especially when deep water running, as it's a totally different sensation to jogging. You feel almost weightless, due to the buoyancy of the water, and your legs and arms seem to move in slow motion. Additionally, your breathing feels different, as the water presses in all around you. However, it's worth giving it a go, as the benefits far outweigh any odd feelings you may experience at first. It may be worth finding a DWR class to get your technique right from the outset, or you can just pick up some instructional articles and video online. Water running is particularly good for the elderly, overweight people and cardiac patients, although it's suitable for anyone and everyone.

Although exercising in water gives 12 times the resistance of exercising in air, you may want to increase the resistance – and burn more calories – by using special water exercise aids, although they are not essential, especially when just starting on a water exercise program. These include aquatics shoes, water weights, fins and paddles. Even foam noodles can be used to create extra resistance and help strengthen limbs and build muscle. Water exercising is a great way to lose weight, build muscle and get fit. Why not give it a go?

Chapter 5
Cycling to Lose Weight and Build Muscle

Cycling, like swimming, is low impact exercise, which means there's less strain on the joints, and you can keep going for longer. While it's not quite so kind to the joints as swimming, it's still a great workout for losing weight and building muscle, and it's enjoyable, which means you're more likely to stick with it. The best exercise in the world is not going to build muscle or help you burn fat and lose weight if you don't do it regularly and often.

Like swimming, cycling is suitable for all ages, abilities and fitness levels. It also has a big advantage over other forms of exercise in that it's also a form of transport. If you're one of those people who have a real aversion to exercise because you'd rather be doing something else, cycling is probably the best form of exercise for you, since it's eco friendly and also useful, in that it gets you where you want to go, while at the same time helping you to get fitter and leaner.

Since cycling doesn't depend on peak performance levels, it's something you can continue to do throughout your life. When you cycle, the saddle and handlebars take the strain off your joints and skeleton, so there's no need to give up cycling because you feel you're too old or too heavy, since around 70% of your body weight is supported by the bicycle. It's a fitness regime you can carry on with for as long you live, if you want to.

The big advantage of cycling is its sheer calorie burning power. It's possible to burn a whopping 670 calories in just 30 minutes, if you can cycle at 15 miles per hour. Even if you can only manage 5 miles an hour, you'll burn roughly 150 calories, depending on your weight and metabolic rate. Talking of metabolism, that essential fat burning activity will stay elevated for several hours following a vigorous cycling session, and that's what you need if you're aiming to lose weight and keep it off. Cycling for just 30 minutes each day will burn off 11 lbs of fat in a year, without undertaking any other exercise.

As for building muscle, cycling falls a little short of swimming in this department, as it particularly develops the muscles in the legs. However, cycling combined with swimming will give your body the all over workout it needs if you're going to lose weight and tone up your body. Cycling is excellent for building strength in the core muscles and the abdominals, and you should see your waist, thighs and butt getting slimmer and more toned as your fitness improves and you are able to put more effort into it. And cycling is a great stamina builder, so not only will you be able to cycle for longer, you'll also be able to do other exercises for longer too, which will help with both weight loss and muscle building.

Consider joining a cycling club – it has numerous advantages over cycling alone. For one thing, you're more likely to be motivated to get on your bike if you commit yourself to club activity. And you'll stretch yourself that little bit further to keep up with your cycling buddies, so you'll get a more thorough workout. Above all, cycling in a noncompetitive group is great fun, and if you enjoy your exercise, you're more likely to stick with it, especially of things get a little difficult on occasion. Then there's the support that only a like-minded group of individuals can give. So, check out the cycling clubs in your area – it's gaining popularity, for exercise, green living and saving on commuting and transport costs, so there's sure to be a cycling club within easy reach of your home.

Cycling is by definition an outdoor activity, and if you can find a cycle path that keeps you away from the roads and the attendant traffic pollution, you'll find your lung capacity increases dramatically, and your heart will become much more effective at pumping blood and oxygen around your body. This makes for improved overall fitness and a reduction in risk factors for heart disease, stroke and diabetes. In fact, recent research figures suggest that people who cycle just 20 miles a week can reduce their risk of heart disease by as much as 50%.

So, cycling is a great way to lose weight, build muscle and burn fat, but if you never learned to ride a bike, or if you're nervous about riding on the roads if there are no cycle paths in your area, there are other ways to get the benefits of cycling without actually going anywhere.

Stationary bike

A stationary exercise bike is a good way to get a full workout in the comfort of your own home or a gym, since it can be used in all weathers and by people of all ages, fitness levels and abilities. A stationary bike is more effective for working on the muscles of the upper body, since there is more scope for changing the exercising position than with a standard bicycle. It's a matter of deciding whether you prefer to exercise indoors or outdoors, and it may be a better option to go for a stationary bike if your co-ordination is poor, or if you are not confident about riding a real bicycle.

Stationary bikes can be upright, which is similar in design and seating position to a bicycle, or recumbent. That means that basically you're sitting with your legs out in front of you and your back supported as if you were sitting on a chair. There are various programs on stationary bikes that will help to vary the intensity of the workout and exercise different muscle groups, so you can get a well rounded workout, although you may find it a little boring compared to riding a bicycle.

You can always alleviate any boredom by listening to music or watching TV as you exercise. However, remember to concentrate on your exercise position and your breathing as you work out.

Spinning

Spinning is the latest exercise craze that's got everybody queuing up to join a spinning class at their local gym or recreation center. Also called studio cycling, it's a high intensity workout aimed at strengthening the heart muscles and toning and slimming the legs. The classes are usually conducted to music and last for around 45 minutes.

The great news is that a spinning class can burn around 500 calories, so it's going to be a big help with weight loss. It can also help with muscle definition, although you may find it rather challenging at first. Many people don't persevere with it, which is a shame, as you can get a great workout through spinning if it's done properly. Look for trademarked spinning classes, so you know you're working with the real thing and not just a cheap – and perhaps dangerous – substitute.

Spinning bikes are something else – the flywheel is weighted for extra resistance and to pick up speed, and the adjustable seat and handlebars give the impression of a conventional cycle. However, you can work at your own pace, since you control everything. And nobody will know if you lag a little behind the others, since everyone finishes at the same time. Nobody knows but you what your level of fitness and pace is, so just keep going, and don't worry about your technique too much until you've got the basics right. Just enjoy, and know that you're helping yourself to lose weight and build muscle without going outdoors. That means you can do spinning all year round.

They say that time passes quickly when you are having fun, and this seems to be true of spinning classes. The instructors are trained to perform and entertain as well as instruct, and many people say it seems no time at all from when they step on their spinning bike until the session ends, and then they feel as if they've really had a great workout, as well as having fun. Exercise should be fun, because if you enjoy it, you're more likely to stick with it, and that's important if you want to stay fit and keep in shape.

Spinning is low impact exercise, so it's ideal for people with arthritis or injuries, who find other types of exercise equipment and other forms of exercise too painful. Because it helps with weight loss, that also helps people with joint problems and injuries, since the less weight you are carrying, the less stress is placed on your joints, and in the long term, this can actually improve your condition and reduce the need for pain relief.

Spinning also gives your abdominal muscles a great workout, particularly if your instructor is on the ball and remembers to remind you about your posture and technique. That's the secret to working the correct muscle groups and getting maximum benefit from your spinning sessions.

Cycling, whether outdoors on a bicycle or indoors on a stationary bike or a spinning bike is a great aerobic workout. It's low impact, so it's suitable for all ages, abilities and fitness levels, and it's something you can do at any time and any age. It's also enjoyable, which means you're more likely to stick with it. As any form of cycling burns lots of calories in a short time, and helps with muscle definition, it's a great aid to weight loss. And because cycling is an activity you're likely to keep up long term, you should be able to keep that weight off once it's gone. What's not to love?

Johnny Fitness

Chapter 6

Dance Your Way to Fitness

Get fit and lose weight by dancing? What's all that about? Well, crazy as it may seem, you can lose weight, get fit and build muscle tone through dance – as long as you pick the right type of dance, that is. A stately waltz around the ballroom floor may be very romantic and enjoyable, but it isn't going to burn calories and fat or build muscles. However, a dance-based exercise class can do just that, and it's still going to be enjoyable too. That's a big plus, because for any exercise to be effective, you need to stick at it, and you're more likely to do that if it's something you enjoy doing.

Here's a round-up of the most popular dance-based exercises around at the moment. There's sure to be a class near you, but if you can't manage to get to a class, there are plenty of videos in the stores and online to help you to lose weight, burn fat and build muscle through dance.

Zumba

Zumba is a relatively modern dance exercise phenomenon. Started by Columbian fitness instructor Alberto Perez back in the 1990s, it's a high energy dance program with a Latin American foundation which incorporates many other forms of dance including salsa, meringue, bhangra, flamenco and belly dancing, among others.

A Zumba class usually lasts for around an hour, and during the session your whole body gets a thorough workout. That means all the major muscle groups are brought into play, so it's great for toning your muscles. And because you burn between 300 and 600 calories during a Zumba class, it's also good for losing weight and fat burning.

Zumba is fast paced and fun, so it's another form of exercise that is a pleasure to take part in, and it's sociable and noncompetitive. It's suitable for all ages and fitness levels, and the Latin beats on which Zumba dancing is based will carry you through the session. You'll wonder where the time went, and will be sorry to get to the end of the class!

Belly dancing

Belly dancing is great fun, and while it doesn't burn as many calories as Zumba – around 300 calories an hour, or maybe a few more – it can help you lose weight if you do it regularly. Look for a class that does a high level of aerobic dancing, because that will help to get your heart rate up and boost the metabolism. Belly dancing also provides gentle strength training, which helps with overall fitness.

Use travelling steps and move your arms in your routines, and this will help to burn calories and boost the metabolism. Keep moving, and maybe practice your shimmy as you do household chores to get the metabolism revving.

You can expect to tone your arms, abdominals and glutes through belly dancing. Most moves originate from the core, so posture is important, and so is repetition of movements. This helps with muscle definition, so get going with the snake arms, belly rolls, figure-of-eights and hip circles. These moves also help with suppleness and flexibility.

If you dance to fast music with a steady beat, you will also be burning fat. That may sound odd but it works. People of all ages can lose weight, burn fat and define their muscles through belly dancing – and men are included in that group too. The best type of belly dancing for weight loss is raqs sharqui. This style of dance includes a lot of arm movements, travelling steps and hip rolls and circle, and these help to tone the muscles as well as burning fat and calories. For best results, and to work all the major muscle groups, try interspersing your belly dancing days with cycling, walking or swimming.

Modern jive

Like belly dancing, modern jive is danced at a fairly fast, steady pace of around 128 – 130 beats per minute (BPM). This will burn between 250 and 500 calories an hour. So it's a fun way to boost your metabolism and burn stubborn fat. It's also a very sociable activity, and once you've got the basics, your posture will improve and your abdominal muscles will strengthen. This immediately makes you look slimmer, fitter and stronger, so you'll feel much better about yourself.

The twists and turns involved in modern jive will work out most of your body's main muscle groups, and you can either learn from a video or DVD, or attend a modern jive class. The class is probably the better option, because as well as having an instructor there to show you the correct techniques and correct your mistakes so you don't injure yourself through poor posture, you'll be mixing with other people.

Modern jive is partner dancing, so it's a lot of fun, and you don't need to be a skilled dancer to do it. It's an excellent way to lose weight, burn fat and tone your muscles while enjoying yourself. And if you enjoy yourself, you'll keep up the exercise.

All forms of dance are excellent exercise as well as being great fun. However, some – such as Zumba, belly dancing and modern jive – are also great for weight loss, fat burning and muscle building. Dance exercise is particularly appropriate for people who do not enjoy regular exercise, or prefer their exercise to be more sociable and fun. It doesn't really matter what you do to exercise, as long as you actually get moving enough to burn calories, so that your metabolism gets a boost and you lose any excess weight and tone muscles. If dance is how you prefer to do that, you've made a great choice, because for you, exercise is never going to be a chore. Rather it will be something sociable that you look forward to with pleasure and anticipation. So, dance the night away, secure in the knowledge that you are helping yourself to better health and fitness at the same time.

Chapter 7

Yoga for Weight Loss and Muscle Development

Yes, you read that right – yoga really can help you to lose weight, burn fat and build muscle. You don't have to throw yourself around the gym, dashing from one set of apparatus to another to get fit. Many people do not realize just how powerful yoga is in helping to sculpt a healthier body.

With yoga, you are lifting weight – but it's your own body weight. As you work your way through the movements and stretches, every muscle group gets a thorough workout. In many yoga poses, such as the shoulder stand and the cobra, you are either lifting or supporting your body weight as you work the muscles, so it is a very effective form of exercise for muscle development. And with this comes a bonus – muscle burns twice as many calories as fat, so it boosts the metabolism, making it easier for you to lose excess weight.

If you have joint problems, yoga is the ideal low impact equivalent to weight training, but it also helps you to align mind, body and spirit in a way that keeps you motivated by making you feel better about yourself. Yoga helps to banish negative energy and thoughts, helping you to attain the right mindset for improving your health and fitness.

Yoga also gives you a great cardio workout, and is excellent for fat burning. Yoga burns between 250 and 350 calories an hour, depending on the style of yoga and the weight of the practitioner. For maximum calorie burning, choose a fast-paced discipline like Ashtanga, Vinyasa or Power yoga. These disciplines are more vigorous, with lots of movement throughout the session, which helps to burn calories and fat.

Another way yoga helps with weight loss is with the mind-body synchronism. Because you are more in tune with your body, you tend to avoid foods that make you feel sluggish. Mostly these are unhealthy foods such as processed foods or items high in refined carbohydrates and sugar, and these are the foods that you need to cut back on in order to shed excess pounds.

Being a holistic exercise discipline, yoga has many fringe benefits, as well as the obvious benefits of losing weight, burning fat and building muscle. It reduces stress, so you are less likely to comfort eat and therefore take in more calories than you can expend through exercise.

For yoga to be effective as a form of weight loss exercise, you need to do at least three 90 minute sessions per week. It makes sense to combine this with other exercise, as yoga may not be able to increase the heart rate enough for cardiovascular health benefits. Maybe you could intersperse your yoga sessions with some cycling, walking or swimming.

The great thing about yoga is that it is suitable for all ages, fitness levels and abilities. Therefore it's an exercise form that is easily accessible to all. The mind/body/spirit element of yoga also helps practitioners to tune into their body's needs, so that they only eat when hungry and avoid unhealthy foods, since they make them feel sluggish and interfere with effective digestion.

The real benefit of yoga is that by focusing on improving the whole lifestyle rather than just on losing weight, people don't become obsessed with their body, and therefore don't develop a negative mindset. It's a different way of looking at things and it works. Recent studies have shown that people who do 30 minutes of yoga each week lost an average of 5 lbs over the 4 years of the study, while those who don't do yoga actually gained an average of 14 lbs over the same period of time. That's 19 lbs average difference in weight between yoga practitioners and the rest.

Yoga is particularly good for helping women develop lean muscle mass rather than the sculpted, ripped muscles men seem to prefer. As muscle burns twice as many calories as fat, this helps tremendously with both weight loss and fat burning. Not only is yoga excellent for helping you to achieve the body you really want, because it changes your focus inwardly, so that your mind and body work in harmony and you are more in tune with your body's needs, it will help you to stay fit and healthy.

To avoid the vicious circle of weight loss and weight gain, you need to rethink your whole life, not just your eating habits and your level of activity. You also need to shed the unhealthy mindset that caused your weight problems in the first place. Yoga can help you to do that, so it's a permanent solution to your weight loss problems, whatever your age or circumstances. Yoga really can help you to be healthy and happy in mind, body and spirit.

Johnny Fitness

Chapter 8

First segment- Beginners Exercises

When it comes to exercising and losing weight, there are certain steps, or procedures, that you have to follow in order to avail maximum benefits. Regardless of whether you are a beginner or an expert, you have to follow the steps and we will look at three different levels of expertise.

In this first segment, we will look at easy exercises that beginners can start performing from immediate effect!

Before we get into the details, there are two important terms that you have to understand. The first one being Reps – that refers to repetitions of the exercises and Sets, which refers to the number of times you must perform the exercise.

Before you start exercising, you must warm up your body in order to awaken it. If you start exercising without warming up your body then you will end up injuring yourself. Let us look at two warm up exercises for beginners.

Warm up 1

The first warm up exercise to take up is known as the march. To perform this exercise:

- Start by standing with a straight back and looking ahead.

- Next, start marching in place.

- Raise your legs as high as possible and move your arms back and forth.

- Continue the process for 5 minutes or until such time as you start feeling warm.

Warm up 2

The second warm up is known as the gentle squats.

- Start by standing straight with your legs joined and hands by your side.

- Now spread your legs just a little and start bending down into a squat.

- You don't have to go all the way down.

- Once you start feeling the burn in your knees you can stop.

Cardio

The very first type of exercise that you must take up after your warm up is cardio exercises. These exercises get your heart rate going and that in turn will help your body start burning fat. So, you have to indulge in some cardio before you get into any of the other exercises. As beginners, it is best for you to take it slow. Don't rush into anything and go about in an orderly fashion.

Cardio exercise 1

The first cardio exercise to take up is skipping.

I'm sure you skipped rope as a child and the same is what you will be doing here.

- Choose a sturdy rope and start skipping.

- You must land softly on your toes.

- If you keep landing on your feet then you will get tired fast.

- If you cannot find a jump rope then simple hold your hands to your side and hold an imaginary jump rope.

- You can skip for 5 minutes or to a count of 200 and stop.

Cardio exercise 2

The next cardio exercise is jumping jacks.
This is a variation of jumping rope and is sure to get your heart racing in no time.

- Start by standing straight with your arms hanging by your side.
- Now jump up and land with your legs apart whilst lifting your hands in the air and joining them on top.
- Jump again and this time, keep your hands by your side and your legs joined.
- Repeat this jumping movement for 5 minutes or to a count of 200.

Cardio exercise 3

The third cardio exercise is the jump squat.

- To perform this exercise, stand in the same position as above by having your feet together and your hands by your side.

- Now jump up and as you land you must get into the squat position.

- You can interlock your fingers and hold your hand out stretched in front of you.

- Jump up again and again land in a squat.

- Ensure that you land softly and are not putting too much pressure under your feet.

- You must do this for 5 minutes or to a count of 30.

Cardio exercise 4

The next cardio exercise is the jump twist. The jump twist will help you exercise both your upper and your lower body.

- Start by standing straight and your arms by your side.

- Now jump up and as you do twist to your right in midair and land straight again.

- On the next jump you must twist to your left and land straight.

- Continue alternating between your jumps.

Cardio exercise 5 (for women)

Women who find it difficult to jump or skip can take up this exercise.

- Start by having a low stool or chair placed in front of you.

- Next, lift both your hands in the air and step on the chair with your right foot and get down quickly.

- Next, step on it with your left foot and get down.

- Keep alternating between your two feet.

It is important to maintain your balance and not fall off from the chair.

As beginners, you can also take up easy cardio exercises such as walking up and down a fleet of stairs, jogging, swimming, cycling etc. As long as it gets your heart rate going it will make for a good cardio exercise.

Weights

Once you are done with your cardio, you must move to lifting weights. Weights will help enhance your cardio workout. It will tone up your body and also define a shape. Let us look at some weights exercises for you to try out.

<u>Weight exercise 1</u>

As a beginner, it is best to pick two dumbbells that weigh 3 lbs. each. The first weight lift will be the simple forearm lift.

- For this, start by standing straight with the dumbbells in your hand.

- Next, turn your fists such that they face you.

- Now holding your elbow in a steady position, lift your forearm towards you.

- Hold in that position for a few seconds and release it back down.

- Repeat again.

- Do 15 reps and 2 sets.

Weight exercise 2

The next exercise to take up is the shoulder lift.

- Start by standing straight and have the dumbbells to your side.

- Now lift it and hold it slightly above your shoulders.

- Lift your arms straight up and then lower it half way before lifting fully up again.

- Next, bring it back full down and then lift it fully up stretched again before bringing it back half way down.

- Do 15 repetitions and 2 sets each.

- If at any time you feel pain or discomfort then stop immediately.

-

Weight exercise 3 (for women)

Most women wish to have a slight curve on their sides but it is quite hard to achieve.

- The best way to bring about the curve is by using weights.

- Start by standing in the neutral position with your legs slightly spread and your hands by your side.

- Hold a dumbbell in each hand.

These are simple weight exercises that you can try and will not require you to put in too much effort. However, if you do find these difficult to take up then you can simply perform the exercises without holding any weight.

Yoga for beginners

Breathing exercise

The first and easiest method is breathing exercises.

- Start by sitting in the lotus pose.

- The lotus pose is where you sit with a straight back, fold your legs and stretch your hands out in front of you.

- Now close your eyes and draw in a few deep breaths.

- Now breathe in at a fast pace such that your breaths are pronounced.

- Breathe out normally and softly.

- Your breaths should originate from your stomach and your stomach muscles should feel the burn.

- Continue for 3 minutes or to a count of 200.

Pavanamuktasan

This exercise is great for your abs and will also improve your digestion.

- Start by lying flat on your back.

- You can lie down on a yoga mat.

- Now fold your legs and bring your knees to your chest.

- You must lift your head and neck up as well and hug your feet using your arms.

- Stay in the position for a few minutes and go back to neutral pose.

- Continue for 5 minutes.

Triangle pose

- To perform the triangle pose start by standing straight.

- Have your legs apart and your hands by your side.

- Now turn to your right and bend down.

- You must attempt to place your left palm on the floor next to your foot.

- Now go back to neutral and bend to your left and place your right palm next to your left foot.

- Go back to neutral pose.

- Do 5 reps on each side.

It is best to perform these yoga poses twice a day for 10 to 20 minutes each. They are level 1 poses and anyone can perform them. Don't worry if you are unable to perform them properly for the first few days. Your body will be quite stiff and take some time to loosen. Once you do loosen your body, these poses will become quite easy to perform.

Chapter 9

Second segment – Intermediate Exercises

In the previous chapter, we looked at easy cardio and weight training exercises that beginners can take up and in this chapter; we will focus on the exercises that intermediators can take up.

Warm up 1

The first warm up exercise to take up is the jogging on spot.

- Start by standing straight and jog on the spot.

- Increase the speed as you go.

- You must jog for a minimum of 5 minutes nonstop until your heart rate rises.

- **<u>Warm up 2</u>**

- The next warm up is the jump kicks.

-

- To perform the jump kicks you must stand straight.

- Now turn to the side and jump up and kick your right leg.

- Now alternate with your left leg.

- Keep alternating your legs and ensure that you are feeling a burn in your entire body.

Calisthenics

<u>Crunches</u>

Crunches are extremely effective in toning up your abs. you can perform them and avail a fit and lean tummy. Here are 2 types of crunches that you can take up.

Regular crunch

The regular crunch is the easiest and best crunch to try out.

- Start by sleeping on the floor and have your hands by your side.

- Now fold your legs and keep them slightly apart.

- Place your arms over your shoulders in a cross manner.

- Now hold your legs glued to the ground and lift your upper torso up.

- You must feel a burn in your lower stomach.

- Go back to neutral and then repeat.

- Do 10 reps and 5 sets of this exercise.

- If you haven't exercised in a while then you can take it a bit slow.

Bicycle crunch

The bicycle crunch is an easy technique yet quite effective.

- Start by lying down on the floor and have your hands by your side.

- Now interlock your fingers and place your hands behind your head.

- Fold your legs and bring it towards your chest.

- Now stretch your right leg out and turn to your left.

- Attempt to touch your left knee using your right elbow.

- Now repeat on the other side.

- Do 15 reps and 3 sets each.

Push-ups

I'm sure you are well aware of the regular push-ups. Although it is a very effective technique, you can enhance its impact by making use of weights.

- To perform this exercise, start by sleeping face down on the ground.

- Ask a helper to place a weight on your lower back.

- Ensure that it is stable and not moving around.

- Now place your palms on the ground and lift your upper body up.

- Assume the plank position and stay there for a few seconds before dropping to the lower push up position.

- Lift your upper body once again.

- You must keep this exercise going for 5 minutes.

Weight exercises

Arms in general
Pinch plates

- Pinch plates are an advanced exercise and will help tone your arms.

- Start by choosing two plates that have quite a bit of weight.

- Pinch them together and hold them in one hand for 30 seconds and then shift it to the other hand.

- Keep shifting the weights back and forth and you must feel a burn in your arms.

Biceps

When it comes to toning your biceps, there is nothing better chin-ups. Chin-ups will help you avail lean biceps and also exercise your entire arm.

- Start by choosing a sturdy rod to perform the exercise.

- Hold your hands apart and ensure that you have enough space to raise yourself up.

- Now use the strength in your upper body to raise yourself up and try to touch the bar using your chin.

- You have to make use of the 2-2 motion where you spend 2 seconds in the upper position and 2 seconds in the lower position.

- Don't worry if you are unable to reach the bar with your chin, with practice you will be able to perfect it.

- You can do 15 reps and 3 sets.

Triceps

The best triceps toning exercise is dips.

- To perform dips start by finding two platforms where one is lower than the other.

- Turn around and place your palms on the higher platform and your feet on the lower platform.

- Now raise your body up using your arms and lower it back down and rise again.

- Continue with this motion for as long as is comfortable.

- You must feel a burn in your upper arms.

It is best to perform these exercises in this particular order itself. You will notice that it is possible for you to push your boundaries every single time and aim higher than before.

Yoga

<u>Downward dog</u>

The downward dog is ideal for intermediate exercisers.

- Start by lying face down on the ground.

- Now place your palms by your side and have your toes resting against the floor.

- Raise your upper body by pushing your palms up and your lower body by pushing your toes up.

- You must end up in a triangular position.

- Hold the pose for a few seconds and release gradually.

- You can repeat this pose 5 to 10 times.

Bridge pose

- To perform the bridge pose start by lying on the floor.

- Now fold your legs try to pull your heels as close to your butt as possible.

- Next, raise your butt from the floor along with your lower back.

- You can then place your arms under your body and interlock your fingers.

- You must create a bridge using your body.

- Remain in the position for a few seconds and release.

- Repeat 10 times.

Shoulder stand

- Start by sleeping on your back.

- Now fold your legs and have your hands by your side.

- Raise your legs in the air and create a 90-degree angle.

- Now use your arms to support your lower back as you further raise your legs.

- All your weight should fall on your shoulders.

- Remain in the position for a few seconds and release.

- You can repeat 5 times.

Plough pose

The plough pose is a continuation of the shoulder pose.

- Assume the shoulder stand and support your lower back with your hands.

- Next, keep pushing your legs back over your head and try to touch the floor behind using your toes.

- This is an advanced pose and don't attempt it if you are not confident.

- Once you touch the floor, remain in the pose for a few seconds.

- Go back to neutral position.

You will get better with these exercises with time.

Chapter 10

Third segment – Expert Level Exercises

Now that we looked at the exercises that intermediaries can take up, we will now look at the ones that experts can take up.

Warm up 1

The best warm up for experts is running a mile.

Start with jogging and then start running.

Once your heart rate is up you can start with your exercises.

Warm up 2

You can run on the treadmill for 30 minutes as well.

Run on the fastest setting and run continuously.

Cross fit training

Cross fit training is a great choice for experts and will help in training the entire body.

Cross fit training has some jargons like WOD which stands for workout of the day and Tabata which refers to doing 20 seconds of an exercise and then taking 10 seconds of rest.

LYNNE

Lynne is the first type of cross fit training that you can take up.

- This exercise calls you to alternate between bench presses and pull-ups.

- Here, you follow a technique known as maximum repetitions. That means that you alternate and perform as many of the exercises as possible within 3 minutes.

- You must do 5 sets each and can take a break of 5 minutes each.

- If at any time you are feeling too tired then you can take a longer break.

- But you must continue with the exercise for as long as possible and push your body if you wish to avail maximum use.

FRAN

The FRAN workout follows a different pattern of exercise. Here, there are no maximum reps and you perform a particular set and then reduce the sets gradually.

- Start with 21 thrusters and 21 pull ups

- You have to put in all your energy and perform the exercises as fast as possible.

- Then, you reduce it to 15 thrusters and 15 pull-ups each.

- Then, you reduce it to 9 thrusters and 9 pull-ups each.

- You can take 2 to 5 minutes break between each and must try to finish all the exercises within 10 to 12 minutes.

These are just two of the cross fit exercises that you can take up but is not limited to just these. You can look up the other exercises and take them up.

Yoga

<u>Matsyasan</u>

Matsyasan is a great exercise to take up and is better known as a cure all.

- Start by sitting on the floor with your legs folded.

- Now lean backwards and sleep on the floor.

- Your legs should remain folded and should be glued to the floor.

- Now raise your head up and push it backwards such that the top of your head lies on the floor.

- You should fixate your gaze behind you.

- Remain in the position for a few seconds and then go back to neutral pose.

- Repeat 5 to 10 times.

Headstand

The headstand is another advanced pose that you can perform only if you are an expert.

- Start by placing your hands on the floor in front of you and interlocking your fingers.

- Next, lift your bottom up and point to the sky.

- Place your head firmly between your interlocked fingers.

- Walk your legs slowly towards your head and lift it up slowly.

- You should balance your entire body on top of your head.

- Remain in the position for as long as is comfortable and then release the pose by slowly placing your legs back down on the floor and go back to neutral.

- You can also take the support of a wall if you wish.

Important notes

- Never take up an exercise without proper warm up; you will end up injuring yourself by doing so.

- Do not exercise on an empty stomach. You will not be able to last the exercise and feel tired.

- Before you take up an exercise regime it is important to inform your doctor. He or she might prescribe some pills to you, which will help your body remain fit.

- If you are already on some form of medication then you must consult your doctor and ask if it is safe for you to continue with the exercise.

Chapter 11

Pre and Post Workout Nutrition

It is extremely important for you to focus on your pre and post workout nutrition. You have to consume foods that are good for your body and those that will supplement your exercise regimen efficiently. In this chapter, we will look at the different foods in detail.

Pre workout nutrition

For your pre workout nutrition, you must consume foods that will give you enough energy to last the workout. We will look at the different pre and post workout ingredients that you have to consume and also a few dishes.

- The first and most important pre workout ingredient to consume is banana. Banana will give you enough energy and will also increase your body's tendency to burn fat.

- The next pre workout ingredient to consume is Greek yogurt. Greek yogurt helps in breaking down the fat in your body.

- It is a good idea to consume oatmeal with a few fresh berries added in.

- Apples too make for great pre workout foods and are sure to get your body ready for a workout.

Recipe 1 - Toast with banana

Calories: 180

Proteins: 2 grams

- Start with a couple of slices of whole wheat bread.

- Toast them without any oil or butter.

- Chop up a few bananas and add to a bowl along with a pinch of cinnamon and give it a toss.

- Now place the banana pieces over the bread and consume.

Recipe 2 - Yogurt smoothie

Calories: 50

Proteins: 12 grams

Start by taking a cup of Greek yogurt and placing it in a blender.

Chop up a few blueberries and some strawberries and add it to the blender.

Whizz until smooth and serve it in a tall glass.

Recipe 3- Oatmeal with veggies

Calories: 70

Proteins: 4 grams

- Start by preparing your oatmeal. Use water to cook it.

- Steam fresh vegetables such as broccoli, corn etc.

- Mix it with the oatmeal along with salt and pepper and consume.

Recipe 4 - Green apple sautéed

Calories: 52

Proteins: 2 grams

- Start by cutting granny smiths into thick wedges.

- Add a knob of almond butter to a saucepan and add in the apple wedges.

- Sauté it for just a few minutes and consume warm.

Post workout nutrition

When it comes to post workout nutrition, you must consume foods that are rich in proteins. Let us look at them in detail.

The first post workout food to consume is lean chicken. You must remove the skin and as much of the visible fat as possible.

Eggs are a great source for proteins and it is mandatory for you to consume them. They are ideal choices for both vegetarians and non-vegetarians.

Chickpeas are loaded with proteins and something like hummus will go a long way in supplementing your body.

- Avocados are packed with nutrition and will help you build a strong body.

- Tuna fish is also a good body booster that you can consume after a workout.

- Skimmed milk along with dark chocolate will help your body regain strength after a tough workout.

Recipe 1 - Spicy chicken grill

Calories: 150

Proteins: 18 grams

- Start by taking two lean chicken thighs and place them in a bowl.

- Add in some Greek yogurt, a teaspoon of cayenne pepper, some sea salt, a teaspoon of black pepper powder, a few cloves garlic and some fresh ginger.

- Give it all a good mix and set it aside for 10 minutes.

- Prepare a grill by heating it.

- Place the chicken thighs on it and cook until the chicken goes pale white.

- Slice the chicken thighs and serve warm.

Recipe 2 - Stuffed eggs with avocado

Calories: 64

Proteins: 5 grams

- Start by hard boiling 4 eggs.

- Meanwhile slice an avocado in half and remove the pit.

- Scoop out the center and add to a bowl.

- Add in some lemon juice, 1-teaspoon mustard, some chili powder and sea salt and give it all a good mix.

- Once the eggs are done, crack them open and slice in half.

- Remove the yolk from the center using a spoon and add it to the avocado mash.

- Mix in well.

- Add the mix to the center of each egg and top it with a cilantro each.

- Consume warm.

Recipe 3 - Salmon sandwich

Calories: 300

Proteins: 20 grams

- Start with two slices of wheat bread.

- Place them on a hot griddle with some almond butter added in.

- Slice the salmon into thin slices and place next to the bread.

- Place the salmon in between the bread and top with mustard and some lettuce leaves.

- You can add in some pepper and salt if you wish to flavor it.

Recipe 4 - Hummus and mixed veggies

Calories: 160

Proteins: 9 grams

- Start by soaking chickpeas in warm water overnight.

- You can also use it straight out of a can.

- Add the chickpeas to boiling water and allow it to go soft.

- Once it does, add to a blender along with some sea salt, some tahini paste or sesame seeds paste, a couple of squeezed lemons and some red chili powder.

- Whizz it until it forms a smooth paste and add in some water if it gets too thick to whizz.

- Cut carrots, cucumbers and bell peppers into thin long wedges and consume with the prepared hummus.

These are the different pre and post workout meals that you must consume on a regular basis. This is just a blue print of the ingredients that you must incorporate. Don't limit yourself to just these and experiment with the ingredients.

With time, you will see that these foods are increasing your body's capacity to undertake the different exercises and also supplementing in the weight loss process.

Johnny Fitness

Chapter 12

BMI and Body Fat

Many people fail to understand the difference between BMI and body fat. The two are not the same. It is easy for you to calculate your BMI using your weight and height information but you cannot self-assess your body fat. You have to visit someone that will assist you with it.

BMI

BMI refers to body mass index. Body mass index is a measurement of your body's mass. It is a measure to see whether you lie within the normal fitness range or is under weight or over weight. There is a very simple calculation that you can do to understand your BMI and that is as follows.

- Start by weighing yourself on a scale.

- You should weigh it in pounds.

- Now multiply your weight by 703.

- Next, measure your exact height in inches, account for any decimals as well.

- Now divide your weight number by your height in inches.

- Once again divide the resultant number with your height in inches and the result is your BMI.

- The ideal BMI for a healthy person is between 18.5 and 24.9. This differs between men and women.

- If you are under 18.5 then it means that you are under weight and need to bulk up. If your weight is over 24.9 then you are overweight. If it is over 30, then you are obese and need to lose a substantial amount of weight.

- You have to measure your weight from time to time and keep a check on your BMI. It is not necessary for you to remain close to the 18 mark. Your BMI can be 20 or 21 and you will still be quite healthy.

- Women are especially advised to be in this range and nothing lower as that can be bad for their bodies.

Body fat

The body fat percentage is another measure of a person's fitness. Here, the total amount of fat that is present inside a person's body is measured. There are special devices for the same and the person is required to sit inside the device and his or her body fat is measured.

- The simple calculation for this technique involves dividing total mass of fat by total body mass.

- Our bodies consist of two types of fats namely the essential body fat and the storage body fat. The former is important for all humans to have in order for the body to function optimally whereas the latter is not something that the body needs.

- The main aim is to reduce the latter as much as possible in order to avail a healthy body.

You can visit a nearby clinic that helps you check your body fat percentage. Some machines are also available in the market now, which will measure it for you but their accuracy is questionable.

Here is a chart for ideal body fat.

TYPE	MEN	WOMEN
ESSENTIAL FAT	10-13%	2-5%
ATHLETES	14-20%	6-13%
FITNESS	21-24%	14-17%
AVERAGE	25-31%	18-24%
OBESE	32%+	25%+

You have to calculate your body fat and then go through this chart to understand whether or not you are within the ideal body fat range. If you have too much fat then you must start exercising and following a lean diet at the earliest. If you continue to remain unhealthy and have too much body fat then you will end up inviting unnecessary illnesses.

Conclusion

While losing weight is challenging, it is possible. With the above exercises, you are sure to lose weight, gain muscle and tone your body the way you want. There is a full range of exercises to suit every level of fitness and ability, and all ages and temperaments.

Some people like to get their exercise outdoors, and for them, walking, running or cycling is best. Others may prefer to hit the gym and train with machines and weights, while for some people swimming is their exercise of choice. Then there are people who don't like exercise, period, but want to lose weight, burn fat and build muscle. For them, maybe dance based exercise or yoga is a better fit.

Whatever type of exercise you decide to take part in, the important thing is that you do it regularly and consistently.

Exercise is not something you just do when you feel like it –
if you want to stay fit and healthy for the rest of your life, you
have to be consistent with your exercise program. Therefore
it makes sense to do something you enjoy, because you are
more likely to keep it going if you enjoy it. The best exercise
in the world will only work if you do it regularly.

Regular exercise, combined with a healthy eating plan is a
guaranteed way to lose weight, burn fat and build muscle.
It's not a quick fix – it takes time and effort, but the results
will be worth it. You will look and feel better, and you will
also reduce your risk of contracting chronic and life-limiting
diseases such as heart disease, diabetes and some cancers.
So take the time to find the right exercise routine for you and
watch those pounds disappear as you achieve the body
you've always wanted and give yourself the priceless gift of
many more years of happy, healthy living.

www.ingramcontent.com/pod-product-compliance
Lightning Source LLC
Chambersburg PA
CBHW040747010626
45792CB00028B/2064